DEDICATION

To the innovators who have the courage to go into the unknown realms of the human psyche.

To the doers, philosophers, and visionaries who work to expand the realm of what is conceivable.

And to each and every reader, may this book encourage you to discover your own great potential.

DISCLAIMER

This book's content is solely intended for educational and informational purposes. It is not meant to be a replacement for expert diagnosis, counsel, or care. Regarding the content's applicability, accuracy, and completeness, the publisher and author make no guarantees or claims.

Regarding any queries or worries about neurological technologies, health, or personal growth, readers are encouraged to speak with knowledgeable experts. Any actions based on the information in this book are not covered by the publisher or the author.

All of the author's ideas are their own, and they may not represent those of any institutions, organizations, or people that are referenced in the book. Unless specifically mentioned, any similarity to actual people, organizations, or technologies is entirely coincidental.

Make responsible and independent use of this book.

Next-Gen Minds

How Neurotechnology is Transforming Human Abilities

Taylor Royce

Copyright © 2024 Taylor Royce

All rights reserved.

CONTENTS

ACKNOWLEDGMENTS..1

CHAPTER 1..1

Overview of Enhancement of Neurology..1

   1.1 Explaining Enhancement of Neurology..1

   1.2 The Development of Neurotechnology and Its Historical Background..2

   1.3 Brain-Computer Interfaces (BCIs) and Their Science.....................5

CHAPTER 2..9

Brain-Machine Interface (BMI) Mechanisms..9

   2.1 Brain-Machine Interfaces That Are Unidirectional..........................9

   2.2 Brain-Machine Interfaces (BBMIs) that are bidirectional...............13

   2.3 Developments in Non-Invasive BMI Technologies..........................16

CHAPTER 3..20

Using Neurological Technology to Improve Cognitive Abilities...............20

   3.1 Improving Cognitive Function: From Recollection to Solving Issues..20

   3.2 Using Wearable Technology to Accelerate Neural Processing.......23

   3.3 Long-Term Cognitive Advantages and Neural Plasticity...............26

CHAPTER 4..30

Using Neuroscience to Improve Human Capabilities.................................30

   4.1 Skill Acquisition's Future..30

   4.2 Using Neurofeedback to Enhance Performance..............................33

   4.3 Incorporating Neurological Development into Expert Education..36

CHAPTER 5...39

Improving Marketing and Consumer Behavior Neurologically............ 39

    5.1 Interpreting Customer Feelings and Thoughts................................39

    5.2 Neuromarketing: Gaining Consumer Insights from Neural Data... 43

    5.3 Consumer privacy and ethical considerations................................45

CHAPTER 6...50

Enhancing Cognitive Function in Gaming and Sports........................ 50

    6.1 Improving Athletic Capabilities..50

    6.2 Neurotechnology as a Competitive Advantage in E-sports and Gaming...54

    6.3 Tracking Performance with Real-Time Cognitive Monitoring........56

CHAPTER 7...61

Neurological Enhancement: Ethical Consequences and Debates......... 61

    7.1 Cognitive Enhancement's Boundaries... 61

    7.2 Neuroethics: Harmonizing Human Rights and Innovation.............64

    7.3 Neurological Enhancement Technology Regulation......................67

CHAPTER 8...71

The Future of Neurological Enhancement: Trends and Predictions.... 71

    8.1 Technological Developments in Neural Interface...........................71

    8.2 Enhancement of Neurology and Artificial Intelligence..................74

    8.3 Prospects for the Future: Beyond Transhumanism........................ 77

CHAPTER 9...82

Improving Neurology in Medicine and Healthcare..............................82

    9.1 Neurotechnologies for Neurological Disease Treatment................ 82

    9.2 Neurological Enhancement and Precision Medicine...................... 86

9.3 Neurotechnology as a Rehabilitation Instrument...........................88

CHAPTER 10..93

Neurological Enhancement: Obstacles and Prospects........................... 93

10.1 Logistical and Technical Difficulties.. 93

10.2 Adoption and Social Acceptance of Neurological Enhancement. 96

10.3 The Way Ahead: Prospects for Development and Innovation...... 99

ABOUT THE AUTHOR... 103

ACKNOWLEDGMENTS

I want to express my sincere appreciation to everyone who helped to make this book possible.

To the scientists, researchers, and inventors who devote their lives to discovering the infinite possibilities of the human mind, your efforts serve as the cornerstone of advancement and motivation for our undertaking.

I want to express my gratitude to my family and friends for their everlasting belief in my goal, support, and encouragement. During this journey, your patience and love have been priceless.

I appreciate my readers' interest and drive to study. Works like this are made possible by your insatiable curiosity.

Finally, I want to express my gratitude for the many hours of work, teamwork, and enthusiasm that went into creating this book. This demonstrates the strength of human potential as a whole.

CHAPTER 1

OVERVIEW OF ENHANCEMENT OF NEUROLOGY

1.1 Explaining Enhancement of Neurology

The use of cutting-edge technology to boost cognitive abilities like memory, concentration, problem-solving, and decision-making is known as neurological enhancement. This emerging discipline pushes the limits of human potential by combining computer science, engineering, and neurology. The ability to interact with and affect brain activity to maximize performance and capabilities is the fundamental component of neurological enhancement.

Fundamentally, neurological improvement entails the intricate yet revolutionary process of reading and decoding brain messages. Brain activity is recorded by technologies such as electroencephalography (EEG) and functional magnetic resonance imaging (fMRI), and sophisticated algorithms evaluate the data to reveal information about cognitive states. With the goal of improving neural performance and efficiency, these findings are subsequently utilized to create therapies that range from direct stimulation of particular brain regions to neurofeedback training.

Neurological augmentation is employed in a variety of contexts in real-world applications:

- **Education and Learning:** Enhancing students' concentration and memory.
- **Workplace Productivity:** Improving innovative problem-solving and decision-making.
- Helping people with brain injuries or cognitive impairments is known as "clinical rehabilitation."

The goal of neurological enhancement is to close the gap between boosted potential and natural capabilities by utilizing the complex mechanisms of the human brain.

1.2 The Development of Neurotechnology and Its Historical Background

Early 20th-century study on the electrical activity of the

brain marked the beginning of the development of neurotechnology. The foundation for comprehending cerebral processes was established by the identification of brainwave patterns, including alpha, beta, and delta waves. With the advent of neurotechnologies like electroencephalography (EEG), brain activity mapping became possible.

Important Turning Points in the Development of Neurotechnology:

1. **1924 – Hans Berger and EEG:** Hans Berger's creation of EEG transformed neuroscience by making it possible to quantify electrical activity in the brain. EEG, which was first applied in therapeutic settings, offered insight into the dynamic processes of the brain.
2. **1960s – The Birth of Brain-Machine Interfaces (BMIs):** The ability to convert brain impulses into useful outputs was shown in early investigations. In order to prepare for BMIs, researchers experimented with using EEG signals to control basic gadgets.
3. **1990s – Neuroimaging Advancements:** High-resolution images of brain activity were made

possible by the development of functional MRI (fMRI) and magnetoencephalography (MEG), which allowed for a better comprehension of cognitive processes.

4. In the 2000s, advancements in neural prosthetics enabled people with motor disabilities to operate robotic limbs with just their thoughts. These developments demonstrated how BMIs can improve the quality of life.

5. **Present Day - Bidirectional Interfaces and AI Integration:** BCIs are more advanced than ever now, incorporating AI to enable bidirectional connection with the brain and more accurate decoding.

As neurotechnology develops further, its uses have spread outside the medical field to encompass professional growth, education, and gaming. Humanity's increasing desire to not only comprehend the brain but also actively improve its functioning is reflected in this progression.

1.3 Brain-Computer Interfaces (BCIs) and Their Science

A key component of neurological augmentation is brain-computer interfaces, or BCIs. Bypassing conventional neuromuscular channels, these systems allow direct communication between the brain and external equipment. Signal acquisition, signal processing, and signal output are the three main parts of BCIs.

Ways that BCIs function

1. Signal Acquisition, which uses tools like intracranial electrodes or EEG to record brain activity. Neural activity, including neuronal firing or oscillatory patterns in certain brain regions, is reflected in the signals.
- **Non-invasive Techniques:** Despite their poor spatial resolution, EEG and near-infrared spectroscopy (NIRS) are commonly employed due to their accessibility and safety.
- **Invasive Techniques:** Although implanted electrodes offer more accurate data, they need surgery, which makes them more appropriate for

clinical settings.

2. Signal Processing: Unprocessed brain signals are complicated and noisy. These signals are filtered, amplified, then decoded into meaningful patterns using sophisticated algorithms.

- Finding particular indicators in the data that are associated with intentions or mental states is known as "feature extraction."
- **Machine Learning**: Artificial intelligence models improve the decoding process, increasing the signal interpretation accuracy.

3. Signal Output: The signals that have been processed are converted into commands for external devices, including exoskeletons, virtual keyboards, or prosthetic limbs. At this point, the user can easily engage with their surroundings.

Brain-Machine Interfaces: Unidirectional vs. Bidirectional

- The main function of unidirectional brain-computer

interfaces (BCIs) is to transmit data from the brain to an external device. A person who is paralyzed, for instance, might utilize a unidirectional BCI to mentally operate a wheelchair.

- **Bidirectional BCIs:** These cutting-edge systems enable two-way brain-to-device connection. They not only interpret brain information but also provide the brain with feedback, including electrical stimulation to enhance memory or motor learning.

BCI Applications:

- **Medical Rehabilitation**: BCIs help patients restore lost functions in cases of stroke, spinal cord injury, or neurodegenerative disorders.
- **Gaming and Virtual Reality:** By enabling users to manipulate avatars or engage with virtual surroundings through thinking, BCIs make immersive experiences possible.
- **Research and Development**: BCIs are used by researchers to investigate how the brain works and create treatments for diseases like depression and epilepsy.

There are difficulties in the field of BCI science. Important factors to take into account include data protection, ethical issues, and the dangers of being overly reliant on technology. However, BCIs have the ability to completely rethink human potential, paving the way for a time when brain improvement will be a fundamental aspect of human growth.

One revolutionary area of human progress is neurological enhancement. Modern neurotechnologies can help society discover new levels of physical and mental performance. Understanding this field's underlying ideas, development across time, and scientific complexities will help us innovate responsibly and make it more widely accessible as we dig deeper.

CHAPTER 2

BRAIN-MACHINE INTERFACE (BMI) MECHANISMS

Advanced systems called brain-machine interfaces, or BMIs, are made to help the human brain and outside equipment communicate. These systems work by recording, deciphering, and converting brain impulses into commands that can operate robotics, computers, and other instruments. Although the mechanisms behind BMIs have changed throughout time, they can be broadly divided into two categories: unidirectional and bidirectional BMIs. Furthermore, non-invasive technology developments are improving safety and accessibility for a larger range of uses. These mechanisms are thoroughly examined in this chapter, which also provides examples of their applications and future possibilities.

2.1 Brain-Machine Interfaces That Are Unidirectional

Systems known as unidirectional brain-machine interfaces

(BMIs) allow data to move from the brain to an external device only. Neural signals are captured, processed, and converted into useful outputs by these interfaces. Unidirectional BMIs are distinguished by the fact that they just serve as output devices and do not give the brain feedback.

The Operation of Unidirectional BMIs

1. Signal Acquisition: Methods like intracortical electrodes for more accurate, invasive data collecting or electroencephalography (EEG) for non-invasive brain signal capture are commonly used in unidirectional BMIs. While intracortical electrodes inserted into the brain measure activity directly from neurons, EEG sensors applied to the scalp pick up electrical activity produced by neurons.

2. Signal Processing: After being recorded, brain signals are filtered and processed to eliminate noise and find significant patterns. These patterns can be decoded with the aid of sophisticated algorithms and machine learning models, which can differentiate between various commands or intentions.

3. Signal Translation: Following processing, the signals are transformed into commands that can be understood by an external device. An order for a robotic prosthetic to grab an object, for instance, may be converted from a thought to move the right hand.

The translated commands allow the user to use their thoughts to control devices such as wheelchairs, computer cursors, and prosthetics.

Unidirectional BMI Use Cases

1. One option for people who have lost limbs or are paralyzed is to employ robotic arms that are controlled by unidirectional BMIs. These prosthetics let users carry out daily functions like shaking hands, opening doors, and grasping things by deciphering signals from the motor cortex.

- **Control and Accuracy**: More dexterous motions, such picking up small objects or typing on a keyboard, are made possible by recent breakthroughs in motor control.

2. Assistive Devices
- **Wheelchair Navigation:** People who are paralyzed can operate powered wheelchairs with just their thoughts. In order to direct the wheelchair's movement, BMIs decipher brain signals related to directional intent (forward, backward, left, and right).
- **Computer Interfaces:** BMIs can be used to operate computer interfaces, allowing people with significant motor impairments to communicate, browse the web, and engage in creative activities like painting.

3. Gaming and Virtual Reality:
- **Immersive Control:** Unidirectional BMIs let users manipulate characters or avatars in virtual worlds, improving the immersion of training simulations or gaming.

These uses demonstrate how unidirectional BMIs are changing people's lives by increasing engagement with the digital world, enhancing mobility, and regaining independence.

2.2 Brain-Machine Interfaces (BBMIs) that are bidirectional

Bidirectional Brain-Machine Interfaces (BBMIs) represent a substantial development over unidirectional systems by providing two-way communication between the brain and external equipment. BBMIs enable both command execution and real-time feedback by letting signals move from the brain to an external device and vice versa.

The Operation of BBMIs

1. Signal Acquisition: Like unidirectional BMIs, BBMIs start by employing electrodes (such as intracortical implants or electroencephalograms) or other sensors to record brain signals.

2. Translation and Signal Processing: The signals that have been recorded are converted into directives for external devices.

3. Feedback Delivery: BBMIs use sensory pathways or direct neural stimulation to deliver sensory feedback to the brain. For instance, feedback sensors on a prosthetic hand can simulate the feeling of touch by sending tactile information to the brain when a user uses it to grip an object.

BBMI Applications

1. Cognitive Feedback in Real Time:
- **Neurofeedback Training:** BBMIs can be used for neurofeedback, which teaches users how to control their brain activity by giving them feedback in real time. This method is used for performance optimization, mental health therapies, and cognitive enhancement.
- **Attention and Focus Training:** BBMIs give people with attention deficit disorders instant feedback on their focus-related brain activity, which helps them learn how to focus better.

2. Sensory Augmentation:

- **Restoring Sensory Function:** BBMIs can help those who have lost or compromised senses regain their sensory experiences. A person who has a robotic arm, for example, can get feedback on the pressure, temperature, or texture of objects they touch.
- **Improving Perception:** In addition to regaining lost abilities, BBMIs can enhance sensory perception by increasing hearing or night vision.

3. Motor Rehabilitation:

- **Recovery after Strokes:** By enabling brain-controlled workouts that offer feedback to improve motor learning and recovery, BBMIs aid in motor rehabilitation. The feedback loop facilitates neuroplasticity, or the brain's ability to reorganize itself for better performance.

5. Learning Optimization:

- **Cognitive Enhancement:** By giving users feedback on their cognitive states and assisting them in improving their memory recall and problem-solving abilities, BBMIs are being investigated as a way to improve learning processes.

Real-time feedback from BBMIs creates new opportunities for improving human-machine collaboration and designing more user-friendly and efficient interfaces.

2.3 Developments in Non-Invasive BMI Technologies

The development of non-invasive methods is one of the most important themes in BMI development. Compared to invasive techniques that necessitate surgical implantation, non-invasive BMIs provide a safer and more convenient option. Recent developments have increased the accuracy and adaptability of non-invasive BMIs, expanding the range of possible uses.

Important Non-Invasive Technologies

1. Transcranial Direct Current Stimulation (tDCS):
- **Mechanism:** tDCS modifies neuronal activity by delivering a small electrical current to the scalp. Depending on whatever area of the brain is stimulated, this can either improve or impair brain

activity.

Applications for tDCS include:
- **Cognitive Enhancement:** tDCS is used to enhance learning, memory, and problem-solving skills.
- **Mental Health:** It has demonstrated potential in the treatment of mood disorders, including anxiety and depression.
- **Motor Skill Training:** tDCS helps musicians and athletes improve their skills and speed up motor learning.

2. Functional Near-Infrared Spectroscopy (fNIRS):
- **Mechanism:** fNIRS measures variations in blood oxygen levels in the brain by using infrared light. This method sheds light on how the brain functions when performing cognitive tasks.

Applications
- **Brain Mapping:** fNIRS is employed in clinical and scientific contexts for non-invasive brain mapping.
- **Wearable sensors:** Real-time brain monitoring outside of lab settings is made possible by portable fNIRS sensors, which are beneficial for sports, education, and workplace efficiency.

3. Electroencephalography (EEG):

- **Mechanism**: EEG uses sensors applied to the scalp to record electrical activity from the brain.

Applications:

- **BCI Systems:** EEG-based BMIs are frequently utilized in cognitive training, gaming, and assistive technologies.
- **Sleep and Stress Monitoring**: EEG tracks brain states to assist manage stress and improve sleep quality.

Non-Invasive BMIs' Potential

1. Safety and Accessibility: Non-invasive techniques remove the dangers of surgery, allowing a wider range of people to obtain BMIs. They are especially useful for applications in consumer electronics, mental health, and education.

2. Scalability: Non-invasive, wearable BMIs may be able to grow to a large scale. This tendency is exemplified by gadgets such as cognitive training applications and headbands that monitor the brain.

3. Future Possibilities:
- **Enhanced Learning Tools:** By instantly adjusting to a learner's cognitive state, non-invasive BMIs could customize educational experiences.
- There is a lot of promise for incorporating BMIs into daily living in the future, from brain-controlled smart homes to cognitive health gadgets.

There are several different and quickly developing mechanisms behind Brain-Machine Interfaces (BMIs). While bidirectional BMIs pave the way for future developments in real-time feedback and sensory enhancement, unidirectional BMIs offer useful tools for improving communication and regaining mobility. BMIs are becoming safer, more widely available, and more incorporated into many facets of life thanks to developments in non-invasive technology. These technologies have the potential to expand human potential and human-machine connection as they develop further.

CHAPTER 3

USING NEUROLOGICAL TECHNOLOGY TO IMPROVE COGNITIVE ABILITIES

The human brain is a remarkable organ that can perform incredible memory, learning, creativity, and problem-solving abilities. New avenues for improving cognitive capacities beyond their inherent constraints have been made possible in recent years by neurological technologies. Wearable technology and neuromodulation are only two of the fast growing options for improving brain function. This chapter explores the workings and possibilities of these technologies, with particular attention to neuroplasticity, memory, problem-solving, and neural processing speed.

3.1 Improving Cognitive Function: From Recollection to Solving Issues

The use of technology to boost mental processes like

memory, learning, problem-solving, and decision-making is known as cognitive augmentation. As our knowledge of the brain expands, so do the strategies for improving its functioning. While natural strategies like education, diet, and mental exercises have historically been used to increase cognitive function, new neurological technology are offering ground-breaking approaches to maximize cognitive abilities.

Memory Enhancement: Deep brain stimulation (DBS) and other technologies are being investigated to improve memory retention and recall. DBS entails implanting electrodes in particular brain areas, like the hippocampus, which is essential for memory formation and retrieval. Although this method is being researched to treat neurodegenerative diseases like Alzheimer's, it also shows promise for improving cognitive function in general.

Case Studies: DBS has demonstrated the ability to help patients with memory impairments in clinical trials. For example, there have been observable gains in memory tests following stimulation of the fornix, a part of the brain linked to memory circuits.

Learning Acceleration: By altering neural activity, neuromodulation methods like transcranial magnetic stimulation (TMS) and transcranial direct current stimulation (tDCS) can promote quicker learning. These non-invasive techniques improve the brain's capacity to take in and remember information by delivering gentle electrical or magnetic pulses to the brain.

Applications: tDCS has been used to enhance the acquisition of motor skills, language, and even mathematics problem-solving. These methods aid in strengthening the neural connections required in learning new tasks by activating the motor or prefrontal cortex.

Executive Function Improvement: Neuromodulation and brain-computer interfaces (BCIs) help improve executive functions, such as planning, decision-making, and impulse control. By focusing on the prefrontal cortex, which is in charge of these higher-order cognitive functions, neurological technology can assist people in becoming more focused, mentally flexible, and capable of making better decisions.

As an illustration, brain-computer interfaces (BCIs) are being developed to treat people with attention deficit disorders by giving them real-time feedback on brain activity. This will help them control their focus and minimize distractions.

People can now maximize their mental performance in both personal and professional circumstances thanks to these cognitive improvement strategies.

3.2 Using Wearable Technology to Accelerate Neural Processing

A potent approach for increasing cognitive processing speed is the wearable neurological gadget. These gadgets, which frequently employ non-invasive techniques, are intended to increase creativity, enhance decision-making, and speed up cognitive activity.

Mechanisms of Action: Neuromodulation methods such as transcranial alternating current stimulation (tDCS), neurofeedback, or tACS are frequently used in wearable technology. By altering the electrical activity of the brain, these techniques improve the effectiveness of neural transmission.

tDCS: tDCS can speed up cognitive processing by reducing the time it takes for neurons to fire by passing a small electrical current through electrodes applied to the head.

tACS: Alternating electrical currents are used to synchronize brain wave patterns, which can enhance reaction times and cognitive coherence.

Instances of Wearable Neurotechnology:
- **Halo Sport:** A neurostimulation headgear that enhances sports performance and motor skill learning with tDCS. It helps musicians and athletes learn complicated moves faster by stimulating the motor cortex.
- The Muse Headband is a wearable EEG gadget that helps users focus and relax by giving them real-time feedback on their brain activity as they meditate.
- The NeuroSky MindWave is a brainwave-sensing headset that enhances concentration and focus. It is

employed in classrooms to assist pupils focus as much as possible.

Uses in Creativity and Decision-Making:

Wearable neurotechnology can be especially helpful in situations requiring fast thinking under pressure. For instance:

- **Military and Emergency Services:** Equipment that improves situational awareness and decision-making speed can be useful for first responders, pilots, and soldiers.
- **Creative Professionals:** To overcome creative blockages and produce original ideas more rapidly, artists, writers, and designers are turning to neurostimulation devices.

Wearable technology is helping people function at higher cognitive levels, cutting down on decision-making time and increasing overall productivity by increasing the speed and efficiency of neural processing.

3.3 Long-Term Cognitive Advantages and Neural Plasticity

The brain's capacity to rearrange itself by creating new neural connections throughout life is known as neural plasticity, or neuroplasticity. Learning, memory formation, and cognitive adaption are all based on this skill. Long-term cognitive benefits can be obtained via neurological technologies that improve brain plasticity, assisting people in maintaining their mental resilience and agility.

The following are some ways that neurological technologies improve neuroplasticity:
- **Brain Stimulation Techniques:** By encouraging the formation of new synaptic connections and strengthening preexisting ones, techniques like tDCS, TMS, and DBS can support neuroplasticity. For instance, by fortifying the neuronal networks involved in movement control, tDCS delivered to the motor cortex can improve motor learning.
- **Brain-Computer Interfaces:** People can learn to control certain brain functions with the aid of BCIs

that offer real-time feedback. This training can improve cognitive capacities over time by causing long-lasting changes in the structure and function of the brain.

Lifetime Cognitive Benefits:
- **Memory Retention:** Improved neuroplasticity promotes improved recall and retention of memories. People can lower their chance of age-related cognitive loss by keeping strong brain connections.
- **Cognitive Reserve:** Neuroplasticity helps the brain maintain its ability to withstand damage from illness, injury, and aging. Higher cognitive reserves enable people to preserve cognitive function and make up for brain loss.

The ability to learn new abilities and adjust to new obstacles throughout life is facilitated by enhanced neuroplasticity. This is especially helpful in a world that is changing quickly and where lifelong learning is crucial.

The following are some useful strategies to improve neuroplasticity:
- **Mental Exercises:** Neuroplasticity can be enhanced

by mentally taxing activities like solving puzzles, picking up new languages, or playing an instrument.
- Regular exercise increases brain-derived neurotrophic factor (BDNF), a protein that aids in the development and upkeep of neurons.
- **Food and Sleep:** A healthy diet full of vitamins, antioxidants, and omega-3 fatty acids, together with enough sleep, promote neuroplasticity and brain health.

Utilizing neuroplasticity, neurological technologies provide a potent means of preserving and enhancing cognitive function throughout time. These technologies promote resilience, mental agility, and lifelong learning by improving the brain's capacity for adaptation and reorganization.

Using neurological technology to improve cognitive capacities is becoming a viable possibility rather than a pipe dream. These technologies are redefining human potential in a variety of ways, from enhanced memory and quicker learning to quicker decision-making and long-term cognitive resilience. The future of cognitive improvement will be significantly shaped by the convergence of neuromodulation, wearable technology, and neuroplasticity-enhancing techniques as research advances. These developments hold the potential to unleash new levels of human performance and well-being in addition to overcoming cognitive constraints.

CHAPTER 4

Using Neuroscience to Improve Human Capabilities

4.1 Skill Acquisition's Future

The Way Neurological Improvement Will Facilitate Quicker and More Efficient Learning

The idea of brain augmentation is transforming the way people learn new skills. To become proficient, traditional learning approaches frequently call for a lot of time and repeated practice. We are on the verge of a day when learning can be expedited by directly interacting with the brain thanks to developments in neuroscience and technology. Traditional learning bottlenecks may be avoided with neurological improvements such as brain-computer interfaces (BCIs), neurochemical therapies, and brain stimulation.

The following are some of the key technologies causing

this change:

- Through non-invasive stimulation of particular brain regions, transcranial magnetic stimulation (TMS) improves neuroplasticity the brain's capacity to reorganize itself and speeds up learning.
- **Neurochemical Enhancers:** Medications that improve cognitive functioning without causing major side effects, such as nootropics, which increase focus and memory retention.
- Devices that directly connect the brain to computers, known as brain-computer interfaces (BCIs), enable quick data transfer and skill programming.

These technologies, for instance, can help musicians improve their ability to perform intricate compositions by fortifying neural connections related to hand-eye coordination, while athletes can utilize them to learn new physical methods. It's possible that within a few decades, the capacity to "upload" knowledge or talents will no longer be confined to science fiction.

Potential Uses in Workforce Development and

Education

Beyond individual growth, neurological enhancement has ramifications for systemic adjustments in workforce training and education. By customizing content delivery to each student's unique brain profile, educational institutions could replace traditional rote learning with individualized neuro-enhanced approaches. Students with learning difficulties could flourish alongside their peers if this democratizes access to education.

Rapid skill development in the workplace made possible by neurological improvement may help close skill gaps in vital industries. Imagine a society in which employees can switch occupations with ease by receiving specialized neural training for new positions. For example:

- **Healthcare:** By using neurofeedback-enhanced simulated environments, surgeons could improve their motor skills and procedural understanding.
- In engineering, experts could become proficient in new design tools or coding languages in a matter of weeks as opposed to years.

- Neural stimulation is a potential tool for artists and designers to access increased creativity and innovation in the creative arts.

Essentially, neurological enhancement is a catalyst for societal advancement as well as a tool for personal development, allowing for a workforce that is more talented and adaptive.

4.2 Using Neurofeedback to Enhance Performance

Optimizing Brain States for Concentration, Focus, and Creativity using Neurofeedback

Through real-time neural signal monitoring, neurofeedback, a state-of-the-art technique based on biofeedback principles, teaches people to control their brain activity. This technique helps people adjust their brain states for peak performance by using sensors to identify patterns in brain waves and software to give feedback in the form of visual or aural signals.

Neurofeedback can target particular brain wave

frequencies in order to:

- By raising beta waves, which are linked to active thinking and problem-solving, you can improve focus and attention.
- Alpha waves, which are associated with feelings of calmness and alertness, are amplified to promote creativity and relaxation.
- High-frequency gamma waves can be modulated to lessen stress and anxiety.

In real-world applications, neurofeedback has helped athletes perform at their best during contests, artists unleash their full creative potential, and executives make better decisions under duress.

The Function of Neurofeedback in Mastering Skills in Various Domains

Neurofeedback is a flexible tool for skill improvement because of its versatility. Through regular neurofeedback treatments, kids with attention difficulties have demonstrated notable gains in their ability to focus and perform well on tests. In a similar vein, neurofeedback helps experts in high-stakes domains like emergency medicine or air traffic control make better decisions in a split second.

Applications of neurofeedback include:

- In order to attain "flow states," where performance feels natural and intuitive, athletes utilize neurofeedback during sports training.
- **Music and Art:** By using neurofeedback to gain increased inspiration, artists and musicians push the frontiers of their trade.
- Neurofeedback is used by executives in corporate leadership to manage stress, stay focused, and enhance strategic thinking.

Its advantages are further democratized by the growing availability of portable neurofeedback equipment, which let consumers practice brain optimization methods in the convenience of their own homes.

4.3 Incorporating Neurological Development into Expert Education

How Neuro-Enhanced Training Methods Can Help Industries Like Medicine, Engineering, and the Arts

The revolutionary potential of neurological upgrades in professional training is starting to be recognized by industries. Improved brain learning could hasten the mastering of intricate diagnoses or surgical techniques in the medical field, where accuracy and experience are crucial. When combined with brain stimulation, simulated worlds enable practical experience without the repercussions of the actual world.

Professionals in engineering, where creativity and problem-solving are critical, can use neuro-enhanced tools to better comprehend and use cutting-edge technologies like robotics and artificial intelligence. Rapid learning and improved spatial reasoning may result in ground-breaking inventions and quicker project completion.

Neuro-enhanced techniques are also bringing forth a

revival in the arts. While performers may enhance their emotional expressiveness by activating brain regions linked to empathy and memory, visual artists can enhance their creativity by tapping into subconscious patterns.

Case Studies of Businesses and Institutions Using Neural Technologies to Enhance Skills

Leading the charge to incorporate neurological enhancement into professional training are a number of trailblazers:

DARPA (Defense Advanced Research Projects Agency):
- DARPA investigates how brain stimulation might improve soldiers' acquisition of vital skills and foreign languages in record time through initiatives such as the Targeted Neuroplasticity Training program.
- The use of virtual reality (VR) in conjunction with neurofeedback is being experimented with by companies such as Accenture and Deloitte to improve employee training, resulting in immersive and highly effective learning environments.

- **Healthcare Training Institutions:** To improve surgeon training, some teaching hospitals are implementing BCIs and VR, which offer real-time feedback on technique and decision-making.

Organizations are enhancing employee satisfaction, cutting training expenses, and improving skill acquisition by integrating these technologies.

The future of human upskilling is in neurological improvement, which gives previously unheard-of chances to boost performance, quicken learning, and transform professional training. The potential is enormous and revolutionary, ranging from neurofeedback tools that improve brain states to industry-wide neural technology applications. As we approach this neurological revolution, the question is not if we will use these technologies, but rather how soon and efficiently we can use them to advance humankind.

CHAPTER 5

IMPROVING MARKETING AND CONSUMER BEHAVIOR NEUROLOGICALLY

5.1 Interpreting Customer Feelings and Thoughts

How Marketers Can Access and Interpret Consumers' Emotional and Cognitive States with the Help of BBMIs

The use of Brain-Based Machine Interfaces (BBMIs) in marketing is transforming how businesses interact and comprehend their customers. BBMIs provide users with previously unheard-of access to their emotional and cognitive states by enabling direct communication between the brain and computer systems. By decoding brain activity, these interfaces can reveal sensations and ideas that are generally overlooked by conventional market research techniques.

Surveys, focus groups, and observational studies have long

been used by marketers to learn about consumer behavior. However, bias, misunderstanding, and the inability to reach subconscious reactions can restrict these approaches. By directly detecting cerebral activity, BBMIs get over these restrictions and provide a more precise and up-to-date evaluation of how customers react to goods, services, and advertisements.

BBMI Applications in Marketing:

- **Mapping Emotions:** Changes in brain activity linked to emotions like excitement, fear, joy, or disgust can be detected by BBMIs. This makes it possible for marketers to measure how consumers feel about ads, product designs, or brand messaging.

- Analysis of Cognitive Load: Marketers can learn how easy or difficult it is for customers to interact with a product or service by using BBMIs, which measure brain activity associated with cognitive processing. This can direct enhancements to product usability and user experience (UX) design.

- **Detection of Subconscious Preference:** Because of societal desirability or ignorance, consumers might not always express their actual desires. By detecting brain markers linked to liking or disliking particular characteristics, BBMIs can uncover these hidden preferences.

The Consequences for Customized Product Development and Marketing

The capacity to decipher emotions and thoughts presents significant prospects for tailored advertising. Marketers may provide highly relevant and tailored content by knowing the preferences and emotional triggers of individual customers. For instance:

- **Personalized Promotions:** Businesses can tailor advertisements to elicit the desired emotional response, such as enthusiasm for a new product or faith in a financial institution, by using real-time brain data.

- **Dynamic Content Adaptation:** By allowing

websites, apps, or virtual reality experiences to dynamically modify content according to users' emotional states, BBMI technology can improve user happiness and engagement.

- **Features of the Tailored Product:** Businesses can prioritize elements in product design that result in greater customer happiness and loyalty by determining which aspects of a product evoke the most positive brain reactions.

- A cosmetics company, for example, may utilize BBMIs to gauge how customers feel about several packaging designs and choose the one that makes them feel the best. According to consumers' cognitive load, an e-commerce platform might also modify its interface in real-time to improve enjoyment and lessen annoyance.

These possibilities are further enhanced by the integration of BBMI technology with machine learning algorithms, which enable ongoing marketing strategy improvement based on changing neural data.

5.2 Neuromarketing: Gaining Consumer Insights from Neural Data

An Overview of Neuromarketing Methods That Assess How the Brain Reacts to Commercials and Goods

By examining how customers' brains react to ads, goods, and brand experiences, the new area of neuromarketing brings neuroscience to marketing. Methods like eye tracking, functional magnetic resonance imaging (fMRI), and electroencephalography (EEG) are frequently employed to assess brain activity and offer insights into how consumers make decisions.

Important Neuromarketing Strategies:

- **The electroencephalogram, or EEG**: EEG uses sensors applied to the scalp to assess electrical activity in the brain. It works well for recording how the brain reacts in real time to stimuli like ads or product displays. EEG can show emotional arousal, engagement, and attention levels.

- **Functional Magnetic Resonance Imaging (fMRI):** fMRI provides fine-grained pictures of brain activity by detecting variations in blood flow throughout the brain. It is helpful in determining which parts of the brain are active during particular marketing activities, such decision-making or brand recognition.

- **Eye-Tracking:** Eye-tracking technology is frequently used in conjunction with neuromarketing to gain insight into visual attention, despite the fact that it is not a direct indicator of brain activity. It assists in identifying the aspects of a product design or campaign that draw the greatest attention.

Case Studies of Businesses Improving Their Marketing Strategies using Neural Data

1. PepsiCo: To test several snack food package designs, PepsiCo used EEG. They chose designs that increased sales after determining which ones elicited the biggest emotional response through the analysis of brain wave data.

2. Hyundai: The automaker employed fMRI to learn how customers responded to various automobile designs. Hyundai improved their designs to better suit consumers' subconscious preferences by tracking brain activity linked to pleasure and desire. This increased their market appeal.

3. Facebook: The social media behemoth used eye tracking and EEG to assess how consumers reacted to various kinds of ads on their network. They were able to maximize engagement by optimizing ad types and locations thanks to their study.

These case studies show how neuromarketing may be used practically to improve advertising tactics, product design, and customer experiences in general. Businesses can use neural data to create data-driven decisions that appeal to their target audiences and eliminate guessing.

5.3 Consumer privacy and ethical considerations

Weighing the Risks of Privacy Invasion Against the

Advantages of Neuro-Enhanced Marketing

Although neurological augmentation has enormous marketing potential, there are serious privacy and ethical issues with it. There is a risk of exploitation, manipulation, and privacy breach while accessing and analyzing customer brain data. It is essential to strike a balance between these advantages and moral issues in order to preserve customer confidence and prevent harm.

Important Ethical Concerns:

- **Conscientious Consent:** Customers need to be properly informed about the collection, use, and storage of their neurological data. Businesses must make sure that participants are aware of the consequences of sharing their brain data and that consent is acquired in a transparent manner.

- **In terms of data security:** Since brain data might disclose personal information about feelings, preferences, and thoughts, it is extremely sensitive. Strong data security measures must be in place to stop misuse or illegal access.

- **Possibility of Manipulation:** It might be possible to influence customers into making decisions that are not in their best interests by deciphering their subconscious inclinations. Transparency must be given top priority in ethical marketing strategies, and vulnerabilities must not be exploited.

The use of brain data for marketing presents both ethical and legal issues.

The laws governing neuro-enhanced marketing are currently being developed. Although they offer principles for data protection, current privacy laws like the General Data Protection Regulation (GDPR) in Europe might not adequately address the particular difficulties presented by brain data. Important legal factors include:

- The problem of who owns neural data the customer, the business that collects it, or a third-party service provider is complicated and calls for precise legal definitions.

- **Cognitive Privacy Right:** According to new debates on cognitive liberty, people ought to be able to manage who can access their brain activity. It could be necessary to amend the law to safeguard this fundamental right.

Ethical Neuromarketing Best Practices:

- **Openness:** Businesses should be transparent about their usage of neuro-enhancement technologies and give concise justifications for the use of brain data.

- **Anonymization of Data:** Neural data should, if feasible, be aggregated and anonymized to preserve privacy.

- **Boards for Ethical Review:** Neuromarketing studies can be supervised by independent ethical review boards to guarantee that participants' rights are upheld and ethical standards are followed.

Businesses can properly utilize neurological enhancement

by tackling these moral and legal issues, making sure that the advantages of neuro-enhanced marketing do not compromise the rights of consumers.

Innovative potential to understand consumer behavior, improve marketing tactics, and develop customized experiences are presented by neurological enhancement. However, there are important privacy and ethical issues with these developments. Marketers may create trust, safeguard consumers, and use brain technologies to create a more moral and successful marketing industry by striking a balance between innovation and accountability.

CHAPTER 6

Enhancing Cognitive Function in Gaming and Sports

Cognitive performance is becoming more and more important in the quest for greatness in gaming and sports. Traditional sports still rely heavily on physical prowess, but it is impossible to overestimate the value of mental clarity, concentration, and judgment. We are entering a time where neurological upgrades can greatly improve performance, giving sportsmen and gamers previously unheard-of advantages, thanks to developments in neurotechnology and brain-machine interfaces (BMIs). This chapter examines the many aspects of optimizing cognitive performance through neurological improvement, looking at its potential, applications, and immediate advantages.

6.1 Improving Athletic Capabilities

While athletes are always looking to enhance their physical

skills, cognitive qualities like focus, decision-making, and response time are equally important for optimal performance. Innovative ways to maximize these cognitive capacities are provided by neurological enhancement treatments, which improve performance on the track, court, or field.

Neurological Enhancement Applications in Sports

Several methods that focus on the brain's functioning to improve cognitive processes necessary for athletic performance are included in neurological enhancement in sports. These consist of:

- **The optimization of reaction time:** For sportsmen participating in sports like basketball, soccer, or sprinting, quick reflexes are essential. Transcranial direct current stimulation (tDCS) is one neurological improvement that can assist fine-tune the brain's motor cortex, increasing the speed at which the brain processes and reacts to inputs.

- **Attention and Focus:** It can be difficult to stay

focused during high-stakes games. By helping athletes enter and maintain ideal brain states (such alpha or beta states) for extended periods of time, techniques like neurofeedback training improve focus and lessen distractions.

- **Efficiency in Making Decisions:** Decisions made in the heat of the moment can decide success or failure. Neurological methods can improve an athlete's capacity to assess circumstances and make the optimal decision under duress by activating parts of the brain involved in decision-making, such as the prefrontal cortex.

Sports Training Brain Stimulation Methods

Numerous methods of brain stimulation are being investigated and used in athletic training regimens. These consist of:

- **Direct current stimulation of the brain (tDCS):** To increase neuronal activity, tDCS applies a small electrical current to particular brain regions.

According to studies, tDCS can boost general cognitive function, lessen fatigue, and improve motor skills.

- The process of transcranial magnetic stimulation, or TMS: TMS stimulates brain nerve cells using magnetic fields. TMS is utilized in sports to improve learning of complex motor tasks, increase hand-eye coordination, and speed up reaction times.

- **The process of neurofeedback training:** Through real-time feedback from electroencephalogram (EEG) sensors, neurofeedback teaches athletes how to regulate their brain waves. This aids athletes in achieving the best possible mental states for concentration, calmness, and performance.

For instance: Neurofeedback has been utilized by Olympic-level shooters and archers to enhance focus and stabilize their hands by preserving a composed and focused condition.

By incorporating these methods into routine training plans,

athletes may be able to fully utilize their cognitive potential and transform the way they prepare.

6.2 Neurotechnology as a Competitive Advantage in E-sports and Gaming

Professional gaming and e-sports have become extremely popular, with players vying for millions of dollars in prizes. In this fiercely competitive setting, every advantage matters. These days, neurotechnology is being used to improve mental endurance, cognitive function, and reaction times, which gives athletes a major edge.

New Developments in Neural Gaming Enhancements

A number of neurotechnologies are being developed to assist e-sports athletes in improving their cognitive abilities:

- **BCIs, or brain-computer interfaces, are:** Direct brain-to-gaming system communication is made possible by BCIs. By avoiding conventional input methods like controllers and keyboards, this technology can assist gamers in improving control precision and lowering reaction latency.

- **Devices for Neurostimulation:** Wearing portable neurostimulation equipment, such as tDCS headsets, during practice sessions can improve brain plasticity and hasten the acquisition of new techniques or abilities.

Gamers can attain the best possible cognitive states for optimal performance by employing equipment that measure and affect brain-wave patterns, such as alpha, beta, and gamma waves. For instance:
- **Alpha Waves:** For a calm but concentrated state.
- **Beta Waves:** To be vigilant and make quick decisions.
- **Gamma Waves:** To improve learning and cognitive processing.

Increasing Mental Stamina and Reaction Times

Games like Counter-Strike, League of Legends, and Fortnite require quick reflexes. Players can reduce their reaction times by milliseconds with the use of neurological enhancement treatments, which can mean the difference between winning and losing. Furthermore, it's critical to sustain mental endurance during extended gaming sessions. Players can manage stress, lessen mental fatigue, and maintain attention for extended periods of time with the aid of strategies like neurofeedback.

Case Study: Neurostimulation devices are being used by some professional e-sports teams as part of their training regimens to improve decision-making and reaction times under duress. These groups report lower burnout rates and more consistent performance.

6.3 Tracking Performance with Real-Time Cognitive Monitoring

Real-time cognitive monitoring offers important insights into a person's mental state in high-stress situations, such as sporting events and video game tournaments. Coaches, trainers, and athletes can track brain activity and make quick modifications to maximize performance by utilizing neurotechnological instruments.

Real-Time Cognitive Monitoring Applications

EEG sensors and other neuroimaging instruments are used in real-time cognitive monitoring to track cognitive states like:

- **Focus Levels:** Assessing a player's or athlete's level of focus at crucial times.
- **Stress and Anxiety:** Recognizing when stress levels increase and putting anxiety management techniques into practice.
- **Detection of Fatigue:** Identifying mental exhaustion before it affects performance and modifying training or competition plans accordingly.

Athletes and Gamers Benefits

- **Instant Feedback:** Adjustments can be made on the fly thanks to real-time data. For instance, coaches can use methods like visualization or deep breathing exercises to help athletes regain attention if they lose it during a competition.

- **Performance Perspectives:** Athletes and gamers can better understand their mental strengths and shortcomings by using detailed cognitive data. Training plans that target particular cognitive difficulties can be customized using this knowledge.

- **Injury Prevention:** Real-time cognitive monitoring in contact sports can assist in detecting indications of cognitive impairment or concussion, allowing for prompt interventions to stop more injuries.

For instance: Real-time cognitive monitoring is being investigated in the NFL to better identify concussions and enable medical personnel to act quickly to ensure player safety.

Cognitive Monitoring Technology and Tools

There are currently a number of tools available for tracking cognitive performance:

- **Wearable EEG equipment**: These lightweight

gadgets provide constant data on brain activity and can be worn while exercising.

- **VR and AR Platforms:** Cognitive monitoring can be integrated into virtual reality (VR) and augmented reality (AR) platforms to replicate high-pressure situations and offer feedback on cognitive performance.

- **Neurofeedback Apps for Mobile Devices:** Apps for gamers and athletes offer feedback and cognitive workouts to improve mental states in real time.

The domains of gaming and sports are being revolutionized by cognitive performance improvement. Athletes and gamers can strengthen their mental stamina, focus, decision-making, and reaction times through neurological upgrades. People are performing at unprecedented levels thanks to methods like neurofeedback, brain stimulation, and real-time cognitive monitoring. The distinction between cognitive and physical training will become increasingly hazy as these technologies develop, leading to a day when achieving top performance requires not only physical skill but also the ability to fully utilize the mind.

CHAPTER 7

NEUROLOGICAL ENHANCEMENT: ETHICAL CONSEQUENCES AND DEBATES

7.1 Cognitive Enhancement's Boundaries

With the potential of enhancing human cognition through the use of cutting-edge technology like nootropic medications, brain-computer interfaces (BCIs), and genetic changes, the idea of cognitive enhancement has recently transformed from a theoretical concept to a quickly growing sector. These developments present previously unheard-of chances to enhance cognitive function in general as well as memory, attention, and problem-solving skills. But they also bring up important moral questions regarding the limits of human improvement and the possible repercussions of exceeding the bounds of natural cognition.

Enhancing human cognition has significant ethical

ramifications since it calls into question long-held beliefs about the integrity of the human experience, the essence of human identity, and the idea of justice. The distinction between "normal" human functioning and "enhanced" skills can be muddled by cognitive enhancement technology, raising new concerns about what it means to be human. With the use of these technologies, people may be able to develop cognitive capacities that are well above those of the general population, creating a new class of "superhumans." Because people who have access to these improvements might be able to exceed others in their personal lives, careers, and even schooling, this raises questions about societal injustice.

The question of fairness lies at the heart of the controversy concerning cognitive enhancement. There is a chance that these technologies will make already-existing social injustices worse if they are made broadly accessible. Access to augmentation technology may be more widespread among those in privileged or wealthy situations, giving them an unfair edge over others. This might cause society to become even more stratified, with those who are more fortunate having disproportionate access to prosperity and opportunities while those who are less fortunate are left behind. Justice and the possibility of further entrenching inequality in social mobility, work, and education are called into question by this situation.

Additionally, there are worries that cognitive improvement could lead to a genetic divide. If it is possible to genetically modify or improve specific cognitive qualities, people who opt out of such upgrades may be severely disadvantaged. This might result in a society that is split along cognitive abilities as well as economic class in the future, with those who are enhanced holding influential and powerful roles and those who are not enhanced possibly being excluded.

The argument about the limits of cognitive augmentation touches on fundamental philosophical considerations regarding human nature in addition to fairness and inequity. Is it moral, for instance, to modify human cognition in a way that could radically alter our identities as individuals? If we start altering our thoughts to the extent that we go beyond our inherent boundaries, will we still be able to maintain our humanity? These are difficult issues that test our conceptions of identity and individual liberty and go to the core of what it is to be human.

7.2 Neuroethics: Harmonizing Human Rights and Innovation

The ethical, legal, and societal ramifications of developing neurotechnologies, such as cognitive enhancement, have given rise to the topic of neuroethics. It is crucial to make sure that innovation is balanced with respect for human rights and the preservation of individual autonomy as these technologies continue to advance at an accelerated rate. Significant issues about privacy, informed consent, and the possibility of coercion are brought up by the use of neural technologies; these issues need to be properly taken into account while designing and implementing these technologies.

One of the cornerstones of bioethics is informed consent, which is especially important when discussing neurological enhancement. People must be completely aware of the risks, advantages, and possible long-term effects of the technology in order to make an informed decision about whether to have cognitive enhancement treatments done.

This entails being aware of the enhancement's immediate impacts as well as any possible negative ones, like personality changes, cognitive biases, or long-term health hazards. Developers and medical professionals need to make sure people are given all the information they need and aren't coerced into choices that don't fit with their interests or values.

The problem of autonomy the freedom of individuals to make decisions regarding their own lives and bodies lies at the core of the neuroethical debate. Technologies for cognitive improvement have the potential to significantly alter people's cognitive abilities, which raises questions about whether they could impair their capacity for autonomous decision-making. Will people still be able to make choices that represent their actual wants and interests if they can be "enhanced" to become more focused, intelligent, or efficient, or will outside influences like social norms or business interests influence their cognitive capacities? This begs the question of whether using augmentation technologies compromises an individual's autonomy, especially in light of potential outside pressure to live up to social norms regarding success or intelligence.

Furthermore, it is impossible to overestimate the role that developers, marketers, and policymakers play in making sure that these technologies are used in an ethical manner. It is ethically required of developers of cognitive enhancement technologies to make sure that the best interests of its consumers are taken into consideration while designing their products. This entails managing possible hazards, guaranteeing security, and being open and honest about the constraints and possible outcomes of their goods. It is also the duty of marketers to refrain from presenting irrational or coercive narratives about cognitive development, as this may lead people to seek improvements that they do not completely comprehend or that do not fit with their beliefs.

The legislative framework pertaining to cognitive enhancement is greatly influenced by policymakers. They have to strike a balance between the necessity of innovation and the defense of individual liberties and the avoidance of exploitation. Laws must be established, for instance, to protect against the possible abuse of cognitive enhancement technology, such as in the workplace, where employers may coerce workers into getting cognitive improvements in order to fulfill performance standards or stay competitive. To guarantee that the advantages of cognitive enhancement are realized without jeopardizing human rights or dignity, policies that support openness, responsibility, and equity must be developed.

7.3 Neurological Enhancement Technology Regulation

The importance of regulatory bodies in guaranteeing the safety, effectiveness, and equity of these technologies is growing as the area of neurological enhancement expands. The particular difficulties presented by these new technologies, which frequently entail intricate relationships between biology, technology, and ethics, must be taken into consideration while designing regulatory frameworks.

The safety of cognitive enhancement technology is one of the main issues that regulatory organizations are concerned about. Despite the fact that many of these technologies offer substantial advantages, nothing is known about how they will affect the body and brain in the long run. The usage of brain implants, nootropic medications, or genetic alterations, for instance, may have unanticipated repercussions that affect a person's health, happiness, or cognitive abilities. Before these technologies are made generally available, regulatory agencies must make sure they go through extensive testing and clinical trials to evaluate their efficacy and safety.

Efficacy is another important consideration in addition to safety. It must be demonstrated that cognitive enhancement technologies provide users with observable advantages, such as better learning capacities, more productivity, or better cognitive performance. However, because the impacts of cognitive enhancers might differ based on the person, the technology, and the situation, efficacy is not always easy to quantify. To set precise efficacy requirements and make sure that customers aren't duped by inflated promises or unproven technology, regulators must collaborate closely with academics and developers.

Perhaps the most difficult part of regulating neurological enhancement technology is the fairness issue. As was previously said, these technologies have the potential to worsen already-existing disparities, especially if only specific groups have access to them. The distribution and use of enhancement technologies must be free from discriminatory practices, and regulatory organizations must guarantee that these technologies are available to everyone, irrespective of socioeconomic background. Policymakers also need to consider how cognitive augmentation might lead to a new kind of social stratification, in which elites or the rich would be the only ones able to access improved cognitive capacities.

The development of comprehensive legislation and regulations pertaining to cognitive enhancement is still in its early stages, and much work needs to be done. To guarantee that these advancements are applied sensibly, morally, and equitably, control of neurological enhancement technologies will undoubtedly be essential. By striking a balance between innovation and human rights, safety, and equity, we can maximize the potential of new technologies while preserving people's dignity and well-being.

The ethical ramifications and disputes surrounding neurological enhancement are discussed in this chapter, emphasizing the intricate relationship between regulation, autonomy, justice, and technical progress. Significant ethical issues are raised by the quick development of cognitive enhancement technologies, however these issues can be resolved while guaranteeing that the advantages of these technologies are distributed fairly and responsibly with careful thought and regulation.

CHAPTER 8

THE FUTURE OF NEUROLOGICAL ENHANCEMENT: TRENDS AND PREDICTIONS

8.1 Technological Developments in Neural Interface

Recent years have seen a fast advancement in neural interface technology, particularly brain-machine interfaces (BMIs), which present intriguing opportunities for improving cognitive function and integrating the brain with external equipment. These technologies are anticipated to develop into increasingly complex, smooth, and generally available systems as we move forward, potentially completely altering the way people communicate with one another and with technology. The next generation of neural interfaces promises to progress beyond the current constraints, enabling more advanced capabilities such as real-time cognitive augmentation, mind-controlled gadgets, and even thought-driven communication.

The miniaturization and integration of the technology will be one of the major developments in the field of neural interfaces. Nowadays, a lot of BMIs necessitate the dangerous and invasive surgical implantation of electrodes into the brain. However, non-invasive or minimally invasive techniques may be developed in the future, enabling safer and more effective neural interface integration. Wearable technology, such patches or headsets, might be used for these interfaces, which would enable smooth communication between the brain and outside equipment without requiring surgery. This will greatly increase neural technologies' accessibility and make them available to a far wider range of people.

Another important consideration in the development of future neural interfaces will be their seamlessness. Neural interfaces will become easier to operate and require less user input or external equipment as they advance. Future BMIs, for instance, would allow people to operate gadgets or complete activities simply by thinking, doing away with the need for conventional input techniques like voice commands, touchscreens, and keyboards. Beyond personal gadgets, this degree of integration might enable people to communicate with smart homes and other networked spaces via straightforward cognitive instructions. Imagine having complete control over your home's lighting, temperature, entertainment, and security systems with just your thoughts a genuinely personalized and easy-to-use smart home experience.

Neural interface technology has the potential to significantly influence autonomous vehicles as well. It is not difficult to envision a future in which drivers (or passengers) may use their brains to control an automobile's systems, steering it with just a thought. Direct brain-to-vehicle communication made possible by BMIs may improve driving and facilitate easier, more effective navigation. Neural interfaces may also be utilized in the creation of driverless cars, in which the artificial intelligence of the vehicle would speak to the user's brain to comprehend their preferences, emotional moods, or cognitive load, enabling a more responsive and customized ride.

A variety of other industries, such as healthcare, education, and entertainment, will also see the integration of neural tech into daily life. Neural interfaces, for example, might be used in medical settings to track brain activity and identify neurological illnesses like Parkinson's or Alzheimer's disease early on, before symptoms appear. By tracking students' brain waves and modifying content delivery according to their cognitive state, educators can design individualized learning experiences that maximize learning outcomes. These are but a handful of the ways that brain interface technology has the potential to greatly improve and enrich our daily lives in the future.

8.2 Enhancement of Neurology and Artificial Intelligence

Artificial intelligence (AI) is being used more and more into the creation and use of neurological upgrades as neural technologies develop. The potential for developing intelligent systems that can react to and interact with brain activity in ever-more-complex ways is increased by the convergence of AI and neurotechnology. The benefits of these technologies could be amplified by the synergy between AI and neurological enhancement, opening up new avenues for enhancing cognitive function, customizing experiences, and maximizing interactions between humans and machines.

One of the most exciting potential for the future of AI and neurological enhancement is the creation of intelligent neuroprosthetics. Artificial intelligence (AI) systems that continuously learn from brain activity and adjust to each person's own cognitive patterns may power these gadgets, which directly connect with the brain. AI might be used, for instance, to improve the functionality of a neuroprosthetic device, like a communication system or memory help for people with neurological problems. The AI might predict demands and modify the device's features to offer a more efficient and customized experience by learning from the user's brain activity.

Another promising field is the integration of AI in cognitive enhancement. Neural interfaces and AI systems could complement each other to enhance cognitive function. AI might, for example, track a user's brain activity in real time and offer suggestions or help with tasks like problem-solving, memory, and concentration. AI has the potential to develop customized cognitive training programs in the future that adjust according to a user's brain waves, improving brain health and the efficacy of cognitive enhancement therapies.

Furthermore, the application of AI could amplify the effects of neurological upgrades by optimizing the method in which neural devices interact with the brain. Large volumes of brain data, for instance, might be analyzed by AI algorithms to find connections and patterns that the human eye could miss. The functionality of neural improvements might then be improved using this data, guaranteeing that the user is getting the most out of them. AI may thus function as a force multiplier, enhancing the accuracy and effectiveness of cognitive upgrades.

AI may potentially play a major part in mental health applications in the future of neurological enhancement and brain-computer interfaces. By examining patterns of brain activity, AI-powered BMIs may be able to identify symptoms of stress, worry, or depression, offering early intervention and real-time mental health management support. In order to enhance well-being, these systems could not only offer therapeutic interventions like cognitive behavioral therapy (CBT) or mindfulness exercises, but also modify the surroundings (such as lighting and sound) according to the user's mental state.

Essentially, the combination of artificial intelligence (AI) with neurological augmentation has the potential to greatly increase the capacity of the human mind, pushing the envelope of what is conceivable and opening up new avenues for cognitive development and personal development.

8.3 Prospects for the Future: Beyond Transhumanism

The long-term prospects of transhumanism, the scientific and philosophical movement that promotes the use of technology to improve the human body and mind, are becoming more and more pertinent as neural technologies develop. According to transhumanism, people will eventually be able to overcome their biological limitations and discover new possibilities for superhuman abilities, immortality, and human evolution. The ability to "upgrade" the brain in previously unthinkable ways makes neural enhancement technologies, in particular, a crucial part of this goal.

The quest for immortality is among the most radical concepts connected to transhumanism. With the use of neural augmentation technology, it is feasible that the human brain might be kept or even augmented permanently. In theory, people could "live" forever in a virtual world, unencumbered by the limitations of biological aging, thanks to technologies like mind uploading, which entails putting a person's consciousness into a digital format. Although this idea is still theoretical, the speed at which neurological technologies are developing raises the prospect that the preservation or improvement of the human mind may one day become a reality.

The quest for superhuman abilities is another long-term objective of transhumanism. Through the use of neural augmentation technology, people may be able to develop superhuman-level cognitive talents, including greater memory, quicker learning, and better problem-solving skills. When a person's cognitive ability exceeds that of the typical human brain, they may develop superintelligence, which could result in the emergence of a new class of people with exceptionally high levels of intelligence. The notion that technology may be used to "upgrade" the human brain presents significant philosophical and ethical problems, especially those pertaining to access, inequality, and the meaning of humanity.

The possibility of humans to "upgrade" the brain has significant philosophical implications. On the one hand, the possibility of prolonging human life and improving cognitive capacities could have enormous advantages, including better quality of life, the elimination of neurological disorders, and the discovery of previously unrealized intellectual potential. However, new technologies may also cast doubt on the veracity of human experiences and essential facets of human identity. The development of a new type of human being one that is not constrained by the biological limitations of the past may result from cognitive enhancement technologies that enable people to transcend their inherent limitations. The ethics of "playing God," the future of human nature, and the effects of such drastic alterations on society at large are all brought up by this.

There is no denying that transhumanism and brain enhancement is a contentious concept with broad ethical, intellectual, and cultural ramifications. However, it might get harder to distinguish between what is technologically improved and what is human as long as technological improvements persist. It will be crucial to carefully assess the implications of these technologies as we go closer to this new frontier, making sure that they are applied sensibly and in a way that advances humankind as a whole.

In conclusion, the field of neurological enhancement has a bright future ahead of it, one that will be greatly influenced by developments in brain interface technology, the fusion of neurotechnology and artificial intelligence, and the pursuit of transhumanist objectives. These technologies raise important ethical, philosophical, and sociological issues that need to be addressed as we proceed, even if they have the potential to drastically alter human cognition. In order to maximize human potential while maintaining the integrity and dignity of what it means to be human, it will be essential to strike a balance between innovation and accountability as we investigate the possibilities of emerging technologies.

CHAPTER 9

Improving Neurology in Medicine and Healthcare

9.1 Neurotechnologies for Neurological Disease Treatment

Millions of people worldwide suffer from neurological illnesses, which are among the most difficult medical problems. Debilitating conditions that cause cognitive decline, physical disability, and a reduced quality of life include post-traumatic stress disorder (PTSD), Parkinson's disease, and Alzheimer's disease. The potential for neurotechnologies to provide ground-breaking treatments is growing along with our understanding of the brain. The use of tools and methods to alter or improve brain activity is known as neurotechnology, and it is being investigated more and more as a potential treatment for a variety of neurological conditions.

The treatment of Alzheimer's disease, a neurodegenerative

condition that causes memory loss, cognitive decline, and ultimately loss of independence, is one of the most promising medical uses of neurotechnology. There are currently few options for treating Alzheimer's disease, and they mostly concentrate on symptom relief rather than treating the underlying causes. Recent developments in neurostimulation and brain-machine interfaces (BMIs), however, are raising the prospect of more potent treatments. For instance, by stimulating particular brain regions to increase neuronal activity, transcranial magnetic stimulation (TMS) has demonstrated promise in reducing cognitive symptoms in Alzheimer's patients. According to one study, TMS helped patients with early-stage Alzheimer's disease with their memory and cognitive function, which suggests that focused neurostimulation could help delay the illness's progression and enhance quality of life.

Neurotechnology is also making progress in the treatment of Parkinson's disease, a degenerative condition that impairs movement control. The loss of dopamine-producing neurons in the brain causes tremors, stiffness, bradykinesia (slowness of movement), and postural instability in Parkinson's disease patients. Deep brain stimulation (DBS) is one of the most promising neurotechnological treatments for Parkinson's disease. In DBS, electrodes are inserted into particular brain regions that control movement, and electrical pulses are used to stimulate these regions. It has been demonstrated that this method greatly lowers motor symptoms and enhances Parkinson's patients' quality of life. Treatment is becoming more individualized and efficient thanks to recent developments in DBS technology, such as closed-loop systems that modify stimulation in real time based on the patient's brain activity.

Neurotechnologies are also showing promise in the treatment of post-traumatic stress disorder (PTSD), which affects many veterans and trauma survivors. PTSD can be quite resistant to conventional kinds of therapy and is typified by intrusive memories, hyperarousal, and emotional numbness. Techniques such as neurofeedback and neuromodulation are becoming promising for treating PTSD. Studies have demonstrated that neurofeedback, which teaches patients to control their own brain activity, can lessen PTSD symptoms by retraining the brain to switch from hyperaroused to more balanced patterns. Transcranial direct current stimulation (tDCS), which involves applying a little electrical current to the scalp to alter brain activity and lessen PTSD symptoms, has also being investigated as a possible treatment. Clinical trials have demonstrated the potential of these therapies, which may give PTSD sufferers fresh hope.

Numerous case studies demonstrate how well neurostimulation works to treat these and other neurological conditions. DBS, for example, dramatically enhanced motor function and decreased tremors in a Parkinson's patient who had not responded to treatment, according to a case study published in The Lancet Neurology. Similarly, even in the latter stages of Alzheimer's, a study published in Neurotherapeutics revealed that TMS treatment significantly improved cognitive function in people with the illness. These incidents highlight how neurotechnologies can revolutionize the treatment of neurological conditions that have long resisted traditional medical interventions.

9.2 Neurological Enhancement and Precision Medicine

The future of neurological enhancement is significantly impacted by the expanding field of precision medicine, a healthcare strategy that considers individual genetic, environmental, and lifestyle factors. Precision medicine has the ability to completely change the way we treat neurological disorders and cognitive enhancement by customizing treatments to each patient's unique needs and traits.

The potential to personalize cognitive enhancements according to unique neurological and genetic profiles is one of the most important developments in precision medicine. Treatments for neurological disorders used to be mainly one-size-fits-all, with little regard for each patient's particular biological composition. But because to developments in genetic sequencing and neuroimaging technology, medical professionals may now obtain comprehensive data regarding a patient's genetic predispositions as well as the shape and function of their brain. Personalized medicines with fewer adverse effects and more efficacy can then be created using this information.

For instance, scientists are investigating the potential of genetic markers to predict which patients are most likely to respond to particular treatments in the case of Alzheimer's disease. Certain genetic differences may make patients more receptive to specific pharmacological therapy or neurostimulation approaches, enabling more focused and efficient interventions. Similar to this, genetic testing can be used to tailor therapies for Parkinson's disease, with some genetic profiles reacting better to particular types of medicine or deep brain stimulation.

Precision medicine may make it possible to customize cognitive enhancement tools in the field of neurological enhancement in order to maximize brain function for each individual. Brain-computer interfaces (BCIs), for instance, which enable users to operate external equipment with their thoughts, may be tailored to each person's cognitive strengths and limitations. These interfaces might adjust in real time to the user's brain activity, offering tailored input or stimulation that improves memory retention, learning, or cognitive performance. Precision medicine may be able to fully utilize neurological technologies by customizing these improvements, enhancing cognitive function and brain health in ways that are tailored to the individual requirements of each patient.

Furthermore, precision medicine for neurological enhancement relies heavily on pharmacogenomics, the study of how genes influence an individual's reaction to medications. For instance, genetic testing may be used to determine which drugs or treatments have the best chance of enhancing cognitive function or reducing symptoms in people with neurological conditions. This method reduces the possibility of negative side effects or ineffectiveness by guaranteeing that patients receive the best treatment possible depending on their genetic profile.

9.3 Neurotechnology as a Rehabilitation Instrument

Additionally, neurotechnology is becoming more and more significant in rehabilitation, especially for people recuperating from brain injuries, strokes, or other neurological impairments. Cognitive or motor function is frequently lost when the brain is damaged or injured, as is the case with a stroke. Although the brain can recover to some extent, this process is frequently sluggish and unfinished. This rehabilitation process is being accelerated and improved by neurotechnologies, especially brain-computer interfaces (BCIs) and neuroprosthetics, giving patients hope when they may otherwise face permanent incapacity.

For instance, by connecting the brain directly to external devices and avoiding injured brain regions, brain-computer interfaces (BCIs) can assist stroke victims in regaining their motor function. For instance, a stroke victim who is unable to move a leg could utilize a brain-computer interface (BCI) to operate an exoskeleton or robotic prosthesis. The patient can restore some motor control by using their thoughts to manipulate the prosthetic device thanks to this direct brain-to-device communication. This can eventually aid in brain rewiring and function restoration in the impacted area, promoting physical healing.

Neurofeedback is another type of neurotechnology used in rehabilitation; it trains patients to control their brain activity, so helping them restore cognitive function. Real-time brain wave monitoring and feedback that teaches the patient how to alter their brain activity is known as neurofeedback. Patients recuperating from brain injuries have found success with this method, which enhances memory, concentration, and other cognitive abilities. Following traumatic brain injury (TBI), neurofeedback has been demonstrated to significantly increase cognitive recovery, enabling patients to restore lost abilities and enhance their quality of life.

The use of neurostimulation techniques as rehabilitation aids is also being investigated, including transcranial direct current stimulation (tDCS). In order to modify brain activity, tDCS applies a small electrical current to particular brain regions. In patients with brain damage, this has demonstrated promise in enhancing speech, memory, and motor skills. tDCS has the ability to activate brain areas related to cognitive or motor control, which can hasten rehabilitation and improve recovery results.

Neurotechnology is also used in rehabilitation through the employment of assistive devices and robotic exoskeletons.

With the use of a brain-computer interface (BCI), these technologies allow people with significant motor impairments to do things that they otherwise would not be able to. Robotic exoskeletons, for instance, may enable people with severe strokes or spinal cord injuries to stand, walk, and carry out other tasks, providing both physical therapy and a psychological boost by enhancing their sense of freedom.

All things considered, neurotechnology has great promise as a rehabilitation tool, helping patients regain their independence and regain lost functions following neurological impairments. The recovery and rehabilitation of people with brain injuries, strokes, and other neurological disorders will depend more and more on these technologies as they develop.

Neurological enhancement has the potential to completely transform medicine and healthcare by providing tailored cognitive boosts, better rehabilitation results, and innovative treatments for a variety of neurological conditions. It is obvious that neurotechnologies will be crucial to healthcare in the future as research and development in this area progresses, enhancing the quality of life for those with neurological disorders and stretching the limits of human cognitive and physical abilities. But when these technologies develop further, it will be crucial to strike a balance between their amazing potential and moral issues, making sure they are applied sensibly to the good of everybody.

CHAPTER 10

Neurological Enhancement: Obstacles and Prospects

10.1 Logistical and Technical Difficulties

A distinct set of technical and logistical challenges arises in the creation and implementation of efficient and scalable neurological augmentation technologies. These technologies are still in their infancy and include neuroprosthetics, neurostimulation devices, and brain-machine interfaces (BMIs). Even though these devices have the potential to transform the way we treat neurological illnesses and improve cognitive function, a number of challenges need to be addressed before they can be routinely used.

Achieving signal accuracy is one of the main obstacles in the development of neurological enhancement technologies. Technologies such as BMIs need to be highly accurate at capturing and interpreting brain activity in order to work well. With billions of neurons interacting with one another via electrical impulses, the brain is an extraordinarily complex organ. One major technical challenge is accurately recording and decoding these signals in real-time, especially in non-invasive devices like electroencephalograms (EEG). For example, current EEG-based BMIs frequently have poor resolution and precision, which might lead to sluggish or inaccurate device control. Despite providing more accuracy, invasive devices come with a number of hazards, such as tissue injury, infection, and bodily rejection.

Another significant issue with several neurological enhancement technologies is their invasiveness. Although neurological illnesses like Parkinson's disease and stroke recovery have showed promise with technologies like deep brain stimulation (DBS) and neuroprosthetics, they require surgical implantation, which carries hazards. The creation of non-surgical, less invasive methods for brain augmentation is still of utmost importance. However, the effectiveness and capacity to target deep brain areas are still limited by even minimally invasive devices, such as those that use transcranial magnetic stimulation (TMS) or transcranial direct current stimulation (tDCS). Furthermore, repeated sessions are generally necessary for these technologies, making them unsuitable for widespread use, particularly in domestic settings.

Another major issue with neurological enhancing devices is their long-term use. The long-term effects of these devices on the brain are still mostly unknown, as is the case with any technology that directly interacts with the human body. For instance, long-term usage of neurostimulation devices may cause neural adaptation, in which the brain gradually loses its sensitivity to the stimulation. Concerns over the safety and effectiveness of long-term use have also been raised by the potential for adverse effects such headaches, cognitive tiredness, or personality changes. To guarantee that these gadgets can be used sustainably to improve neurological functions over time, research into their long-term consequences is essential.

The scalability of neurological enhancing technology presents another logistical problem. Even while a lot of these technologies exhibit potential in small-scale studies or clinical settings, it can be difficult to translate them into generally available and reasonably priced solutions. The majority of neurotechnologies available today are costly, need specific tools, and must be operated by highly qualified specialists. Costs must decrease and the technologies must be made simpler, possibly even to the point where they can be utilized in domestic settings, before they can be widely adopted. Along with technology advancements, this also entails modifications to the regulatory approval procedures and healthcare infrastructure.

10.2 Adoption and Social Acceptance of Neurological Enhancement

A number of issues, such as ethical considerations, public perception, and cultural attitudes toward brain enhancement, will impact the social acceptance and adoption of neurological enhancement technologies as they develop. It is both intriguing and contentious to consider the idea of using technology to improve human intelligence or physical capabilities. These technologies have the potential to help people overcome neurological abnormalities and improve their quality of life, but they also bring up a number of issues that may prevent them from being widely accepted.

The fear of over-dependence on technical advancements is one of the main issues. People may be concerned that using technology to improve their physical or mental capabilities may result in a loss of their feeling of autonomy or personal agency. For instance, the notion of improving memory or learning skills through a brain-machine interface may make people wonder if they might still function normally without these gadgets. There is a worry that we might rely too much on technology to do things that our own natural cognitive processes used to be able to do.

Another major social worry is the concept of unnatural brain upgrades. The idea of using technology to change the brain's natural state may make many people uneasy. Cultural, religious, or philosophical views that regard human intellect as sacred or untouchable are frequently the source of this uneasiness. According to this perspective, brain improvements could be viewed as an instance of unnatural interference with the mind, which could have unforeseen repercussions. Some groups of people may object to the idea of "playing God" by modifying brain processes or even aiming for superhuman capacities through technology.

Concerns about neurological enhancement technology' accessibility and equity are also quite important. These very costly and highly skilled medical technologies have the potential to worsen already-existing healthcare disparities. There may be widening gaps in cognitive and neurological capacities between various socioeconomic classes if just a small percentage of people can buy or use these technologies. This would bring up ethical questions regarding whether efforts should be made to enable equitable access for everyone or whether technical advancements should be kept for the privileged.

The marketing of these technologies and the stories that surround them will shape the public perception of neurological enhancement. These technologies might be more widely accepted if they are marketed as instruments for enhancement and empowerment. However, public opposition may prevent their acceptance if they are perceived as a threat to personal freedom or as a possibility for exploitation. Policymakers, neurotechnologists, and ethicists must interact with the public, listen to their worries, and provide them frank, open information on the advantages, dangers, and moral ramifications of these technologies.

10.3 The Way Ahead: Prospects for Development and Innovation

Notwithstanding the difficulties, neurological enhancement has a bright future full of opportunities for development and expansion. Opportunities for startups, researchers, and companies seeking to develop next-generation neurotechnologies are abundant in this field. Improvements in genetic research, neuroimaging, and artificial intelligence are opening the door to more individualized, efficient, and widely available brain enhancement technologies. Innovations in neurological disease treatment, rehabilitation, and cognitive enhancement may result from the confluence of these domains.

There are several prospects in neurological enhancement for startups and entrepreneurs. Demand for increasingly specialized, user-friendly gadgets that address certain requirements, like memory improvement, stress reduction, or mental health management, will increase as the market for neurotechnologies expands. Furthermore, wearable neurotechnologies, such neurofeedback headbands or brainwave-sensing gadgets, may become commonplace and enable people to maximize cognitive function in their everyday lives. Although there is a sizable market for these consumer-focused devices, their development will necessitate creative approaches to device design, user experience, and pricing.

The area of neurological enhancement presents researchers with fascinating chances to investigate the nexus of neuroscience, technology, and medicine. New avenues for comprehending mental health and cognitive processes are made possible by the capacity to modify and improve brain function. Researchers can investigate the potential applications of neurotechnologies to cure a range of neurological conditions, such as depression and Alzheimer's disease, or to improve cognitive function in healthy people. Furthermore, it will be crucial for neurotechnologists, ethicists, and policymakers to work together to make sure that these developments are in line with moral standards and social demands.

Cross-disciplinary and cross-industry cooperation will also be necessary for the future. Addressing the moral, legal, and societal issues surrounding neurological enhancement will require cooperation between neurotechnologists, ethicists, and policymakers. Legislators must, for instance, create rules governing the safe application of neurotechnologies, making sure that they are usable, efficient, and do not present excessive risks to people. The application of these technologies will be heavily influenced by ethical considerations, particularly when it comes to matters like privacy, autonomy, and informed consent. The future of neurological enhancement and the equitable and responsible distribution of its advantages will be determined in large part by these debates.

In summary, neurological enhancement technologies face significant but manageable challenges. Realizing the full potential of these technologies will require overcoming technological obstacles, tackling social issues, and encouraging collaborative innovation. A future where cognitive and neurological function can be maximized for improved health, performance, and quality of life is promised as long as research and development in the field of neurological enhancement continues.

ABOUT THE AUTHOR

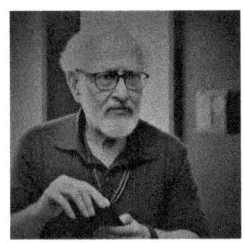

Author and thought leader in the IT field Taylor Royce is well known. He has a two-decade career and is an expert at tech trend analysis and forecasting, which enables a wide audience to understand complicated concepts.

Royce's considerable involvement in the IT industry stemmed from his passion with technology, which he developed during his computer science studies. He has extensive knowledge of the industry because of his experience in both software development and strategic consulting.

Known for his research and lucidity, he has written multiple best-selling books and contributed to esteemed tech periodicals. Translations of Royce's books throughout the world demonstrate his impact.

Royce is a well-known authority on emerging technologies and their effects on society, frequently requested as a speaker at international conferences and as a guest on tech podcasts. He promotes the development of ethical technology, emphasizing problems like data privacy and the digital divide.

In addition, with a focus on sustainable industry growth, Royce mentors upcoming tech experts and supports IT education projects. Taylor Royce is well known for his ability to combine analytical thinking with technical know-how. He sees a time when technology will ethically benefit humanity.

www.ingramcontent.com/pod-product-compliance
Lightning Source LLC
Chambersburg PA
CBHW071036240526
45469CB00006BD/2232